# LOW CARB VEGETARIAN TYPE 2 DIABETES COOKBOOKS FOR BEGINNERS

*Delicious and Easy-to-Follow Plant-Based Recipes for a Healthy Low-Carb Lifestyle, Specifically Designed for Type 2 Diabetes Management*

**By Mia Bennett**

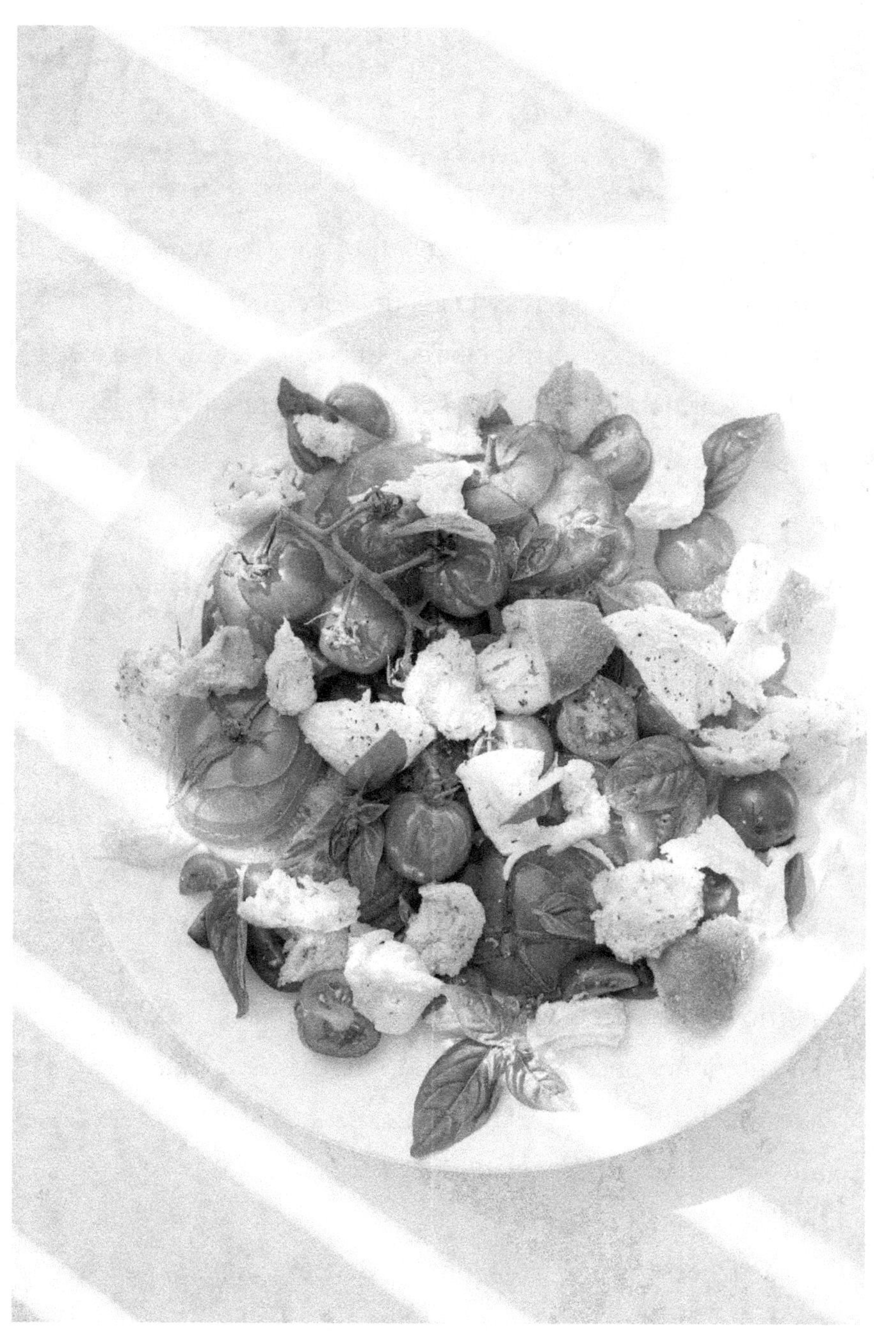

# TABLE OF CONTENTS

## Chapter 5: Snacks and Appetizers ..................... 87

# INTRODUCTION

I magine your body is a bustling city, and blood sugar is the fuel that keeps everything running smoothly. In Type 2 Diabetes, this delivery system gets a bit wonky. The body becomes resistant to insulin, the hormone that ushers sugar into cells for energy. This can lead to a traffic jam of sugar in the bloodstream, causing a host of health concerns.

Fear not, fellow citizen! Diet is a powerful tool to manage Type 2 Diabetes. Enter the low-carb vegetarian approach, a delicious and effective way to keep your blood sugar in check. Here's how to navigate this path and transform your kitchen into a diabetes-fighting haven.

## The Power of Plants: Why Low-Carb Vegetarian Works

Refined carbohydrates like white bread and sugary treats are notorious blood sugar spikers. A low-carb vegetarian diet replaces these with a symphony of colorful vegetables, filling legumes, and nuts. These plant powerhouses are packed with fiber, which slows down sugar absorption, keeping your blood sugar levels cruising smoothly. Plus, you'll get a generous dose of vitamins, minerals, and healthy fats – all essential for overall well-being.

## Pantry Staples for the Savvy Diabetic Vegetarian

Let's stock your kitchen with the essentials! Here's your vegetarian low-carb dream team:

- **Leafy Green All-Stars:** Kale, spinach, and Swiss chard are the base of many a delicious meal. They're low in carbs and brimming with vitamins A, C, and K.
- **Rainbow Riot**: Stock up on a vibrant array of bell peppers, broccoli, mushrooms, and eggplant. These add flavor, fiber, and essential nutrients to every dish.
- **Legume Love:** Beans, lentils, and chickpeas are protein powerhouses packed with fiber. Think hearty chili, lentil stews, or chickpea curries.
- **Nutty Delights:** Almonds, walnuts, and flaxseeds are healthy fat champions. Sprinkle them on salads, yogurt bowls, or enjoy a small handful as a snack.
- **Flavor Boosters:** Don't forget the spices! Herbs like basil, oregano, and cilantro add pizzazz without the carbs. Garlic, ginger, and turmeric are anti-inflammatory superstars.

# Planning and Prep: Your Recipe for Success

Planning your meals is key to staying on track. Here are some tips:

- **Batch Cook Like a Boss:** Cook a big pot of lentil soup or a veggie stir-fry on the weekend. Portion them out for quick and healthy lunches throughout the week.
- **Chop Chop Time**: Dedicate a specific time each week to chopping vegetables. Prepping these colorful ingredients in advance makes whipping up healthy meals a breeze.
- **Leftovers are Lifesavers:** Don't toss those leftovers! Repurpose them into creative lunches or dinners. Leftover roasted veggies can be transformed into a frittata, or leftover chili can become a baked potato topping.

# Kitchen Arsenal: Tools for the Diabetic Vegetarian Warrior

Equipping your kitchen with the right tools can make healthy cooking enjoyable and efficient. Here's your starter pack:

- **Sharp Knives:** A good chef's knife and a paring knife are essential for chopping vegetables with ease.

- **Sheet Pans:** These versatile pans are perfect for roasting vegetables, baking tofu, or creating one-pan meals.
- **Food Processor (Optional):** This handy tool can be a time-saver for chopping vegetables, making nut butters, or pureeing sauces.
- **Slow Cooker (Optional):** This is a weeknight lifesaver. Throw in your ingredients in the morning and come home to a delicious and healthy meal.

**Remember**, this journey is yours! Experiment with flavors, explore new vegetarian recipes, and find what works best for you. With a little planning and creativity, you can manage your Type 2 Diabetes, embrace a plant-powered lifestyle, and turn your kitchen into a delicious haven of health.

# Chapter 1: 30 Day Meal Plan

## Week 1

Day 1

- Breakfast: Spinach and Feta Omelette
- Lunch: Grilled Vegetable Salad with Balsamic Dressing
- Dinner: Eggplant Lasagna
- Snack: Guacamole with Cucumber Slices
- Dessert: Avocado Chocolate Mousse

Day 2

- Breakfast: Chia Seed Pudding with Berries
- Lunch: Cauliflower Rice Stir-Fry
- Dinner: Cauliflower Crust Pizza
- Snack: Stuffed Mini Bell Peppers
- Dessert: Almond Flour Brownies

Day 3

- Breakfast: Avocado Toast with Radishes and Chives
- Lunch: Lentil and Vegetable Soup
- Dinner: Stuffed Zucchini Boats
- Snack: Kale Chips
- Dessert: Keto Cheesecake Bites

Day 4

- Breakfast: Greek Yogurt with Nuts and Seeds
- Lunch: Zucchini Noodles with Pesto
- Dinner: Keto Veggie Stir-Fry with Tofu
- Snack: Roasted Chickpeas
- Dessert: Chia Seed Pudding

Day 5

- Breakfast: Cauliflower Hash Browns
- Lunch: Eggplant Parmesan
- Dinner: Creamy Spinach and Mushroom Casserole
- Snack: Veggie Sticks with Hummus
- Dessert: Coconut Flour Cookies

Day 6

- Breakfast: Almond Flour Pancakes
- Lunch: Chickpea Salad with Lemon-Tahini Dressing
- Dinner: Grilled Portobello Mushrooms with Avocado Salsa
- Snack: Almond Butter and Celery Sticks
- Dessert: Berry Crumble

Day 7

- Breakfast: Vegetable Frittata
- Lunch: Broccoli and Cheddar Soup

- Dinner: Ratatouille
- Snack: Zucchini Chips
- Dessert: Lemon Coconut Balls

## Week 2

Day 8

- Breakfast: Tofu Scramble with Vegetables
- Lunch: Spaghetti Squash with Marinara Sauce
- Dinner: Spaghetti Squash Alfredo
- Snack: Cauliflower Buffalo Bites
- Dessert: Chocolate Zucchini Bread

Day 9

- Breakfast: Low Carb Smoothie Bowl
- Lunch: Stuffed Bell Peppers with Quinoa
- Dinner: Thai Coconut Curry with Vegetables
- Snack: Edamame with Sea Salt
- Dessert: Pumpkin Spice Muffins

Day 10

- Breakfast: Cottage Cheese with Cinnamon and Berries
- Lunch: Mushroom and Spinach Stuffed Portobello
- Dinner: Cauliflower Mac and Cheese

- Snack: Cheese and Olive Platter
- Dessert: Raspberry Almond Tart

Day 11

- Breakfast: Portobello Mushroom Cap with Eggs
- Lunch: Greek Salad with Tofu
- Dinner: Grilled Asparagus with Lemon-Garlic Sauce
- Snack: Spinach and Artichoke Dip
- Dessert: Low Carb Chocolate Bark

Day 12

- Breakfast: Keto-friendly Granola
- Lunch: Roasted Veggie Buddha Bowl
- Dinner: Brussels Sprouts with Walnuts and Balsamic Reduction
- Snack: Mini Caprese Skewers
- Dessert: Peanut Butter Cups

Day 13

- Breakfast: Zucchini Muffins
- Lunch: Low Carb Veggie Tacos
- Dinner: Stuffed Acorn Squash
- Snack: Cucumber Roll-Ups with Avocado
- Dessert: Blueberry Muffins

Day 14

- Breakfast: Flaxseed Porridge
- Lunch: Cauliflower Pizza with Veggie Toppings
- Dinner: Broccoli Cheddar Casserole
- Snack: Broccoli Tots
- Dessert: Coconut Macaroons

## Week 3

Day 15

- Breakfast: Cheese and Veggie Stuffed Bell Peppers
- Lunch: Cucumber and Avocado Gazpacho
- Dinner: Roasted Vegetable Medley
- Snack: Stuffed Mushrooms
- Dessert: Chocolate Covered Strawberries

Day 16

- Breakfast: Spinach and Feta Omelette
- Lunch: Grilled Vegetable Salad with Balsamic Dressing
- Dinner: Eggplant Lasagna
- Snack: Guacamole with Cucumber Slices
- Dessert: Avocado Chocolate Mousse

Day 17

- Breakfast: Chia Seed Pudding with Berries
- Lunch: Cauliflower Rice Stir-Fry
- Dinner: Cauliflower Crust Pizza
- Snack: Stuffed Mini Bell Peppers
- Dessert: Almond Flour Brownies

Day 18

- Breakfast: Avocado Toast with Radishes and Chives
- Lunch: Lentil and Vegetable Soup
- Dinner: Stuffed Zucchini Boats
- Snack: Kale Chips
- Dessert: Keto Cheesecake Bites

Day 19

- Breakfast: Greek Yogurt with Nuts and Seeds
- Lunch: Zucchini Noodles with Pesto
- Dinner: Keto Veggie Stir-Fry with Tofu
- Snack: Roasted Chickpeas
- Dessert: Chia Seed Pudding

Day 20

- Breakfast: Cauliflower Hash Browns
- Lunch: Eggplant Parmesan

- Dinner: Creamy Spinach and Mushroom Casserole
- Snack: Veggie Sticks with Hummus
- Dessert: Coconut Flour Cookies

## Day 21

- Breakfast: Almond Flour Pancakes
- Lunch: Chickpea Salad with Lemon-Tahini Dressing
- Dinner: Grilled Portobello Mushrooms with Avocado Salsa
- Snack: Almond Butter and Celery Sticks
- Dessert: Berry Crumble

# Week 4

## Day 22

- Breakfast: Vegetable Frittata
- Lunch: Broccoli and Cheddar Soup
- Dinner: Ratatouille
- Snack: Zucchini Chips
- Dessert: Lemon Coconut Balls

## Day 23

- Breakfast: Tofu Scramble with Vegetables
- Lunch: Spaghetti Squash with Marinara Sauce
- Dinner: Spaghetti Squash Alfredo

- Snack: Cauliflower Buffalo Bites
- Dessert: Chocolate Zucchini Bread

Day 24

- Breakfast: Low Carb Smoothie Bowl
- Lunch: Stuffed Bell Peppers with Quinoa
- Dinner: Thai Coconut Curry with Vegetables
- Snack: Edamame with Sea Salt
- Dessert: Pumpkin Spice Muffins

Day 25

- Breakfast: Cottage Cheese with Cinnamon and Berries
- Lunch: Mushroom and Spinach Stuffed Portobello
- Dinner: Cauliflower Mac and Cheese
- Snack: Cheese and Olive Platter
- Dessert: Raspberry Almond Tart

Day 26

- Breakfast: Portobello Mushroom Cap with Eggs
- Lunch: Greek Salad with Tofu
- Dinner: Grilled Asparagus with Lemon-Garlic Sauce
- Snack: Spinach and Artichoke Dip
- Dessert: Low Carb Chocolate Bark

Day 27

- Breakfast: Keto-friendly Granola
- Lunch: Roasted Veggie Buddha Bowl
- Dinner: Brussels Sprouts with Walnuts and Balsamic Reduction
- Snack: Mini Caprese Skewers
- Dessert: Peanut Butter Cups

Day 28

- Breakfast: Zucchini Muffins
- Lunch: Low Carb Veggie Tacos
- Dinner: Stuffed Acorn Squash
- Snack: Cucumber Roll-Ups with Avocado
- Dessert: Blueberry Muffins

Day 29

- Breakfast: Flaxseed Porridge
- Lunch: Cauliflower Pizza with Veggie Toppings
- Dinner: Broccoli Cheddar Casserole
- Snack: Broccoli Tots
- Dessert: Coconut Macaroons

Day 30

- Breakfast: Cheese and Veggie Stuffed Bell Peppers

- Lunch: Cucumber and Avocado Gazpacho
- Dinner: Roasted Vegetable Medley
- Snack: Stuffed Mushrooms
- Dessert: Chocolate Covered Strawberries

# Chapter 2: Breakfast Recipes

Breakfast is often hailed as the most important meal of the day, particularly for those managing their health, including individuals with type 2 diabetes. These recipes are designed to be both nutritious and delicious, focusing on low-carb options that support stable blood sugar levels. Whether you prefer savory or sweet, there's something here to kickstart your day with energy and balance.

## Spinach and Feta Omelette

Ingredients:

- 2 eggs
- 1 cup fresh spinach, chopped
- 1/4 cup crumbled feta cheese
- Salt and pepper to taste

Instructions:

1. In a bowl, whisk the eggs until well combined.
2. Heat a non-stick skillet over medium heat and spray with cooking spray.
3. Pour the whisked eggs into the skillet and let them cook for a minute or two.

4.  Add chopped spinach and crumbled feta cheese evenly over one half of the omelette.

5.  Fold the omelette in half and cook for another minute until the cheese melts and the eggs are fully cooked.

6.  Season with salt and pepper to taste.

Nutrition Information (per serving):

- Calories: 250
- Protein: 18g
- Carbohydrates: 4g
- Fat: 18g
- Fiber: 1g
- Sugar: 2g
- Portion Size: 1 omelette

## Chia Seed Pudding with Berries

Ingredients:

- 1/4 cup chia seeds
- 1 cup unsweetened almond milk
- 1/2 teaspoon vanilla extract
- Stevia or sweetener of choice (optional)
- Fresh berries for topping

Instructions:

1.  In a bowl, mix chia seeds, almond milk, vanilla extract, and sweetener (if using). Stir well.
2.  Let it sit for 10 minutes, then stir again to break up any clumps of chia seeds.
3.  Refrigerate overnight or for at least 2 hours until the mixture thickens into a pudding-like consistency.
4.  Serve chilled, topped with fresh berries.

Nutrition Information (per serving):

- Calories: 180
- Protein: 6g
- Carbohydrates: 18g
- Fat: 10g
- Fiber: 12g
- Sugar: 2g
- Portion Size: 1 serving

## Avocado Toast with Radishes and Chives

Ingredients:

- 1 slice of low-carb bread (such as almond flour bread)
- 1/2 ripe avocado
- 2-3 radishes, thinly sliced

- Fresh chives, chopped
- Salt and pepper to taste

Instructions:

1. Toast the slice of low-carb bread until golden brown.
2. Mash the avocado and spread it evenly on the toasted bread.
3. Top with thinly sliced radishes and chopped chives.
4. Season with salt and pepper to taste.

Nutrition Information (per serving):

- Calories: 200
- Protein: 5g
- Carbohydrates: 12g
- Fat: 15g
- Fiber: 7g
- Sugar: 1g
- Portion Size: 1 slice of toast

## Greek Yogurt with Nuts and Seeds

Ingredients:

- 1/2 cup Greek yogurt (unsweetened)
- 1 tablespoon mixed nuts (almonds, walnuts, pecans), chopped

- 1 tablespoon mixed seeds (chia seeds, flaxseeds), ground
- Fresh berries for topping
- Optional: drizzle of honey or sweetener of choice

Instructions:

1. Spoon Greek yogurt into a bowl.
2. Sprinkle chopped nuts and ground seeds over the yogurt.
3. Add fresh berries on top.
4. Optionally, drizzle honey or sweetener over the yogurt mixture.
5. Mix gently before serving.

Nutrition Information (per serving):

- Calories: 220
- Protein: 15g
- Carbohydrates: 12g
- Fat: 12g
- Fiber: 4g
- Sugar: 6g
- Portion Size: 1 serving

# Cauliflower Hash Browns

Ingredients:

- 2 cups cauliflower rice (fresh or frozen)
- 1/4 cup grated Parmesan cheese
- 1 egg
- 1/2 teaspoon garlic powder
- Salt and pepper to taste
- Cooking spray or olive oil for cooking

Instructions:

1. If using fresh cauliflower, pulse in a food processor until it resembles rice.
2. Microwave the cauliflower rice for 4-5 minutes or until tender. Let it cool.
3. In a bowl, combine cauliflower rice, Parmesan cheese, egg, garlic powder, salt, and pepper.
4. Heat a non-stick skillet over medium heat and spray with cooking spray or add a little olive oil.
5. Form the cauliflower mixture into patties and place them in the skillet.
6. Cook for 3-4 minutes on each side until golden brown and crispy.
7. Serve hot.

Nutrition Information (per serving):

- Calories: 150
- Protein: 10g
- Carbohydrates: 8g
- Fat: 8g
- Fiber: 3g
- Sugar: 3g
- Portion Size: 2 hash browns

## Almond Flour Pancakes

Ingredients:

- 1 cup almond flour
- 2 eggs
- 1/4 cup unsweetened almond milk
- 1 tablespoon melted butter or coconut oil
- 1/2 teaspoon baking powder
- 1/2 teaspoon vanilla extract
- Optional: stevia or sweetener of choice to taste

Instructions:

1. In a bowl, whisk together almond flour, baking powder, and optional sweetener.

2. In another bowl, beat eggs and add almond milk, melted butter or coconut oil, and vanilla extract. Mix well.

3. Combine wet and dry ingredients until smooth.

4. Heat a non-stick skillet over medium heat and lightly grease with butter or oil.

5. Pour batter onto the skillet to form pancakes (about 1/4 cup batter per pancake).

6. Cook until bubbles form on the surface, then flip and cook until golden brown on both sides.

7. Serve warm with your favorite toppings.

Nutrition Information (per serving):

- Calories: 280
- Protein: 10g
- Carbohydrates: 8g
- Fat: 24g
- Fiber: 4g
- Sugar: 1g
- Portion Size: 3 pancakes

## Vegetable Frittata

Ingredients:

- 4 large eggs

- 1/2 cup diced bell peppers (any color)
- 1/2 cup chopped spinach
- 1/4 cup diced onions
- 1/4 cup diced tomatoes
- 1/4 cup shredded cheese (cheddar or mozzarella)
- Salt and pepper to taste
- Cooking spray or olive oil

Instructions:

1. Preheat the oven to 350°F (175°C).
2. In a bowl, whisk the eggs until well combined. Season with salt and pepper.
3. Heat an oven-safe skillet over medium heat and spray with cooking spray or add a little olive oil.
4. Sautee the diced onions and bell peppers until softened, about 3-4 minutes.
5. Add chopped spinach and diced tomatoes to the skillet and cook for another 2 minutes until spinach wilts.
6. Pour the whisked eggs evenly over the vegetables in the skillet.
7. Sprinkle shredded cheese on top.
8. Transfer the skillet to the preheated oven and bake for 12-15 minutes, or until the eggs are set and the edges are golden brown.

9.  Remove from the oven and let it cool slightly before slicing and serving.

Nutrition Information (per serving):

- Calories: 180
- Protein: 14g
- Carbohydrates: 5g
- Fat: 11g
- Fiber: 1g
- Sugar: 2g
- Portion Size: 1/4 of the frittata

## Tofu Scramble with Vegetables

Ingredients:

- 1/2 block firm tofu, drained and crumbled
- 1/2 cup diced bell peppers (any color)
- 1/4 cup diced onions
- 1/2 cup chopped spinach
- 1/4 cup cherry tomatoes, halved
- 1/2 teaspoon turmeric powder
- Salt and pepper to taste
- Cooking spray or olive oil

Instructions:

1. Heat a non-stick skillet over medium heat and spray with cooking spray or add a little olive oil.
2. Add diced onions and bell peppers to the skillet and sauté until softened, about 3-4 minutes.
3. Add crumbled tofu to the skillet and sprinkle turmeric powder over the tofu. Mix well to combine.
4. Cook for 3-4 minutes, stirring occasionally, until tofu is heated through and lightly browned.
5. Add chopped spinach and cherry tomatoes to the skillet. Cook for another 2 minutes until spinach wilts and tomatoes soften.
6. Season with salt and pepper to taste.
7. Remove from heat and serve hot.

Nutrition Information (per serving):

- Calories: 220
- Protein: 18g
- Carbohydrates: 10g
- Fat: 12g
- Fiber: 4g
- Sugar: 4g
- Portion Size: 1 serving

# Low Carb Smoothie Bowl

Ingredients:

- 1/2 cup unsweetened almond milk
- 1/2 cup frozen berries (such as strawberries, blueberries, raspberries)
- 1/2 small avocado
- 1 tablespoon chia seeds
- Optional toppings: sliced almonds, shredded coconut, fresh berries

Instructions:

1. In a blender, combine almond milk, frozen berries, avocado, and chia seeds.
2. Blend until smooth and creamy, adding more almond milk if needed to reach desired consistency.
3. Pour the smoothie into a bowl.
4. Top with sliced almonds, shredded coconut, and fresh berries.
5. Serve immediately and enjoy!

Nutrition Information (per serving):

- Calories: 250
- Protein: 7g
- Carbohydrates: 18g

- Fat: 17g
- Fiber: 10g
- Sugar: 6g
- Portion Size: 1 bowl

## Cottage Cheese with Cinnamon and Berries

Ingredients:

- 1/2 cup low-fat cottage cheese
- 1/2 teaspoon ground cinnamon
- 1/4 cup mixed berries (such as strawberries, blueberries, raspberries)
- Optional: drizzle of honey or sweetener of choice

Instructions:

1. In a bowl, combine cottage cheese and ground cinnamon.
2. Top with mixed berries.
3. Optionally, drizzle honey or sweetener over the cottage cheese and berries.
4. Mix gently before serving.

Nutrition Information (per serving):

- Calories: 150

- Protein: 15g

- Carbohydrates: 15g

- Fat: 3g

- Fiber: 3g

- Sugar: 10g

- Portion Size: 1 serving

## Portobello Mushroom Cap with Eggs

Ingredients:

- 2 large Portobello mushroom caps

- 2 eggs

- 1/4 cup diced bell peppers (any color)

- 1/4 cup diced tomatoes

- Salt and pepper to taste

- Fresh herbs for garnish (such as parsley or chives)

Instructions:

1. Preheat the oven to 375°F (190°C).

2. Remove the stems from the Portobello mushroom caps and gently scrape out the gills with a spoon.

3. Place the mushroom caps on a baking sheet lined with parchment paper, gill side up.

4. Crack one egg into each mushroom cap.

5. Scatter diced bell peppers and tomatoes evenly around the eggs.

6. Season with salt and pepper.

7. Bake in the preheated oven for 15-20 minutes, or until the egg whites are set.

8. Remove from the oven and garnish with fresh herbs.

9. Serve hot.

Nutrition Information (per serving):

- Calories: 180
- Protein: 14g
- Carbohydrates: 8g
- Fat: 10g
- Fiber: 3g
- Sugar: 5g
- Portion Size: 1 stuffed mushroom cap

## Keto-friendly Granola

Ingredients:

- 1 cup almonds, chopped
- 1 cup pecans, chopped
- 1/2 cup unsweetened shredded coconut
- 1/4 cup sunflower seeds

- 1/4 cup pumpkin seeds
- 1/4 cup chia seeds
- 1/4 cup flaxseeds
- 1/4 cup coconut oil, melted
- 1/4 cup sugar-free maple syrup or sweetener of choice
- 1 teaspoon vanilla extract
- 1/2 teaspoon ground cinnamon
- Pinch of salt

Instructions:

1. Preheat the oven to 300°F (150°C) and line a baking sheet with parchment paper.
2. In a large bowl, combine chopped almonds, pecans, shredded coconut, sunflower seeds, pumpkin seeds, chia seeds, and flaxseeds.
3. In a separate bowl, whisk together melted coconut oil, sugar-free maple syrup (or sweetener), vanilla extract, ground cinnamon, and a pinch of salt.
4. Pour the liquid mixture over the nut and seed mixture, and stir until well combined and evenly coated.
5. Spread the granola mixture in an even layer on the prepared baking sheet.
6. Bake for 25-30 minutes, stirring halfway through, until the granola is golden brown and crisp.

7. Remove from the oven and let it cool completely on the baking sheet.

8. Once cooled, break the granola into clusters and store in an airtight container.

Nutrition Information (per serving):

- Calories: 220
- Protein: 6g
- Carbohydrates: 8g
- Fat: 18g
- Fiber: 5g
- Sugar: 1g
- Portion Size: 1/4 cup

## Zucchini Muffins

Ingredients:

- 2 cups almond flour
- 1/4 cup coconut flour
- 1 teaspoon baking powder
- 1/2 teaspoon baking soda
- 1/2 teaspoon salt
- 1 teaspoon ground cinnamon
- 3 eggs

- 1/4 cup coconut oil, melted
- 1/4 cup sugar-free maple syrup or sweetener of choice
- 1 teaspoon vanilla extract
- 1 cup grated zucchini (excess water squeezed out)
- Optional: 1/4 cup chopped nuts (such as walnuts or pecans)

Instructions:

1. Preheat the oven to 350°F (175°C) and line a muffin tin with paper liners.
2. In a large bowl, whisk together almond flour, coconut flour, baking powder, baking soda, salt, and ground cinnamon.
3. In another bowl, whisk together eggs, melted coconut oil, sugar-free maple syrup (or sweetener), and vanilla extract until smooth.
4. Add the wet ingredients to the dry ingredients and stir until well combined.
5. Fold in grated zucchini and chopped nuts (if using) until evenly distributed.
6. Divide the batter evenly among the muffin cups, filling each about 3/4 full.
7. Bake for 20-25 minutes, or until a toothpick inserted into the center comes out clean.

8. Remove from the oven and let the muffins cool in the tin for 5 minutes before transferring to a wire rack to cool completely.

Nutrition Information (per muffin):

- Calories: 180
- Protein: 6g
- Carbohydrates: 8g
- Fat: 14g
- Fiber: 3g
- Sugar: 1g
- Portion Size: 1 muffin

## Flaxseed Porridge

Ingredients:

- 1/4 cup ground flaxseeds
- 1 cup unsweetened almond milk
- 1/2 teaspoon ground cinnamon
- 1/2 teaspoon vanilla extract
- Optional: stevia or sweetener of choice to taste
- Toppings: fresh berries, chopped nuts, shredded coconut

Instructions:

1. In a small saucepan, combine ground flaxseeds, almond milk, ground cinnamon, and vanilla extract.

2. Heat over medium-low heat, stirring constantly, until the mixture thickens to a porridge-like consistency, about 3-5 minutes.

3. Remove from heat and sweeten with stevia or sweetener if desired.

4. Pour into a bowl and top with fresh berries, chopped nuts, and shredded coconut.

5. Serve warm and enjoy!

Nutrition Information (per serving):

- Calories: 150
- Protein: 5g
- Carbohydrates: 8g
- Fat: 10g
- Fiber: 6g
- Sugar: 1g
- Portion Size: 1 serving

# Cheese and Veggie Stuffed Bell Peppers

Ingredients:

- 2 large bell peppers (any color)
- 1/2 cup cottage cheese
- 1/4 cup shredded mozzarella cheese
- 1/4 cup diced tomatoes
- 1/4 cup diced zucchini
- 1/4 cup diced mushrooms
- 1/4 teaspoon dried oregano
- Salt and pepper to taste
- Cooking spray or olive oil

Instructions:

1. Preheat the oven to 375°F (190°C).
2. Cut the tops off the bell peppers and remove the seeds and membranes.
3. In a bowl, mix together cottage cheese, shredded mozzarella cheese, diced tomatoes, diced zucchini, diced mushrooms, dried oregano, salt, and pepper.
4. Stuff the bell peppers with the cheese and veggie mixture, pressing down gently to fill completely.
5. Place the stuffed bell peppers in a baking dish sprayed with cooking spray or lightly coated with olive oil.

6. Bake for 25-30 minutes, or until the bell peppers are tender and the cheese is melted and bubbly.

7. Remove from the oven and let them cool slightly before serving.

Nutrition Information (per serving - 1 stuffed bell pepper):

- Calories: 180
- Protein: 12g
- Carbohydrates: 12g
- Fat: 9g
- Fiber: 4g
- Sugar: 6g
- Portion Size: 1 stuffed bell pepper

# Chapter 3: Lunch Recipes

For a satisfying midday meal that keeps your energy stable and your taste buds happy, explore these diverse lunch options. Each recipe is crafted to be low carb and vegetarian-friendly, perfect for managing Type 2 diabetes while enjoying delicious flavors.

## Grilled Vegetable Salad with Balsamic Dressing

Ingredients:

- Assorted vegetables (bell peppers, zucchini, eggplant, cherry tomatoes)
- Mixed greens
- Olive oil
- Balsamic vinegar
- Salt and pepper

Instructions:

1. Preheat grill to medium-high heat.
2. Toss vegetables with olive oil, salt, and pepper.
3. Grill vegetables until tender and slightly charred.
4. Arrange mixed greens on a plate, top with grilled vegetables.
5. Drizzle with balsamic vinegar.

6. Serve immediately.

Nutrition Information (per serving):

- Calories: 250
- Protein: 5g
- Carbohydrates: 20g
- Fat: 15g
- Fiber: 8g
- Sugar: 10g
- Portion size: 1 salad

## Cauliflower Rice Stir-Fry

Ingredients:

- Cauliflower rice
- Mixed vegetables (bell peppers, broccoli, carrots)
- Soy sauce (low sodium)
- Sesame oil
- Garlic, minced
- Green onions

Instructions:

1. Heat sesame oil in a large skillet over medium heat.
2. Add minced garlic and cook until fragrant.

3.  Add mixed vegetables and stir-fry until tender-crisp.

4.  Stir in cauliflower rice and soy sauce.

5.  Cook until cauliflower rice is heated through.

6.  Garnish with chopped green onions.

7.  Serve hot.

Nutrition Information (per serving):

- Calories: 180
- Protein: 8g
- Carbohydrates: 15g
- Fat: 10g
- Fiber: 6g
- Sugar: 5g
- Portion size: 1 cup

## Lentil and Vegetable Soup

Ingredients:

- Lentils (green or brown)
- Mixed vegetables (celery, carrots, onions)
- Vegetable broth
- Olive oil
- Bay leaves
- Herbs and spices (thyme, parsley, pepper)

Instructions:

1. Heat olive oil in a large pot over medium heat.
2. Sauté onions, celery, and carrots until softened.
3. Add lentils, vegetable broth, bay leaves, and seasonings.
4. Bring to a boil, then reduce heat and simmer until lentils are tender.
5. Adjust seasoning to taste before serving.
6. Garnish with fresh herbs if desired.

Nutrition Information (per serving):

- Calories: 220
- Protein: 12g
- Carbohydrates: 30g
- Fat: 5g
- Fiber: 10g
- Sugar: 5g
- Portion size: 1 cup

## Zucchini Noodles with Pesto

Ingredients:

- Zucchini, spiralized
- Basil pesto (homemade or store-bought)
- Cherry tomatoes, halved

- Pine nuts
- Parmesan cheese (optional)

Instructions:

1. Heat a small amount of olive oil in a skillet over medium heat.
2. Add zucchini noodles and cook until just tender.
3. Toss with basil pesto until evenly coated.
4. Remove from heat and stir in cherry tomatoes and pine nuts.
5. Garnish with grated Parmesan cheese if desired.
6. Serve warm or cold.

Nutrition Information (per serving):

- Calories: 180
- Protein: 6g
- Carbohydrates: 10g
- Fat: 12g
- Fiber: 4g
- Sugar: 5g
- Portion size: 1 cup

# Eggplant Parmesan

Ingredients:

- Eggplant, sliced into rounds
- Low carb marinara sauce
- Mozzarella cheese, shredded
- Parmesan cheese, grated
- Almond flour
- Eggs
- Olive oil
- Italian seasoning

Instructions:

1. Preheat oven to 400°F (200°C).
2. Dip eggplant slices in beaten eggs, then coat with almond flour mixed with Italian seasoning.
3. Heat olive oil in a skillet over medium heat.
4. Fry eggplant slices until golden brown on both sides.
5. Spread marinara sauce on the bottom of a baking dish.
6. Arrange fried eggplant slices in the dish, layering with marinara sauce and mozzarella cheese.
7. Top with grated Parmesan cheese.
8. Bake for 20-25 minutes until cheese is bubbly and golden.
9. Let cool slightly before serving.

Nutrition Information (per serving):

- Calories: 280
- Protein: 15g
- Carbohydrates: 15g
- Fat: 18g
- Fiber: 5g
- Sugar: 8g
- Portion size: 1 piece

## Chickpea Salad with Lemon-Tahini Dressing

Ingredients:

- Chickpeas (canned, drained and rinsed)
- Cucumber, diced
- Cherry tomatoes, halved
- Red onion, thinly sliced
- Parsley, chopped
- Lemon juice
- Tahini
- Olive oil
- Salt and pepper

Instructions:

1.  In a large bowl, combine chickpeas, cucumber, tomatoes, red onion, and parsley.

2.  In a small bowl, whisk together lemon juice, tahini, olive oil, salt, and pepper to make the dressing.

3.  Pour the dressing over the salad and toss gently to coat.

4.  Adjust seasoning if needed.

5.  Chill in the refrigerator for at least 30 minutes before serving.

Nutrition Information (per serving):

- Calories: 220
- Protein: 10g
- Carbohydrates: 25g
- Fat: 10g
- Fiber: 8g
- Sugar: 5g
- Portion size: 1 cup

## Broccoli and Cheddar Soup

Ingredients:

- Broccoli florets
- Vegetable broth

- Cheddar cheese, shredded

- Heavy cream (or coconut cream for vegan option)

- Onion, chopped

- Garlic, minced

- Butter (or olive oil)

- Nutmeg

- Salt and pepper

Instructions:

1. In a large pot, melt butter over medium heat.

2. Add chopped onion and garlic, sauté until softened.

3. Add broccoli florets and vegetable broth, bring to a boil.

4. Reduce heat and simmer until broccoli is tender.

5. Blend soup until smooth using an immersion blender or transfer to a blender in batches.

6. Stir in heavy cream, cheddar cheese, nutmeg, salt, and pepper.

7. Simmer for another 5-10 minutes until cheese is melted and soup is heated through.

8. Adjust seasoning to taste before serving.

Nutrition Information (per serving):

- Calories: 280

- Protein: 12g

- Carbohydrates: 15g

- Fat: 20g

- Fiber: 5g

- Sugar: 5g

- Portion size: 1 cup

## Spaghetti Squash with Marinara Sauce

Ingredients:

- Spaghetti squash

- Low carb marinara sauce

- Olive oil

- Garlic, minced

- Fresh basil, chopped

- Parmesan cheese, grated (optional)

- Salt and pepper

Instructions:

1. Preheat oven to 400°F (200°C).

2. Cut spaghetti squash in half lengthwise and scoop out seeds.

3. Drizzle cut sides with olive oil and season with salt and pepper.

4. Place squash halves cut-side down on a baking sheet lined with parchment paper.

5. Roast for 40-50 minutes until tender and easily pierced with a fork.

6. While squash is roasting, heat olive oil in a saucepan over medium heat.

7. Add minced garlic and sauté until fragrant.

8. Stir in marinara sauce and simmer for 10-15 minutes.

9. Once squash is cooked, use a fork to scrape the flesh into spaghetti-like strands.

10. Serve spaghetti squash topped with marinara sauce, fresh basil, and grated Parmesan cheese if desired.

Nutrition Information (per serving):

- Calories: 200
- Protein: 5g
- Carbohydrates: 30g
- Fat: 8g
- Fiber: 8g
- Sugar: 12g
- Portion size: 1 cup of spaghetti squash with sauce

## Stuffed Bell Peppers with Quinoa

Ingredients:

- Bell peppers (any color)

- Cooked quinoa

- Black beans (canned, drained and rinsed)

- Corn kernels (fresh or frozen)

- Onion, diced

- Garlic, minced

- Cumin

- Paprika

- Salsa

- Cheddar cheese, shredded (optional)

- Fresh cilantro, chopped

Instructions:

1. Preheat oven to 375°F (190°C).

2. Cut the tops off bell peppers and remove seeds and membranes.

3. In a large skillet, heat olive oil over medium heat.

4. Sauté diced onion until translucent, then add minced garlic and cook until fragrant.

5. Stir in cooked quinoa, black beans, corn, cumin, and paprika.

6. Cook for 5-7 minutes until heated through.

7. Remove from heat and stir in salsa.

8. Spoon quinoa mixture into bell peppers, packing tightly.

9. Place stuffed peppers in a baking dish and cover with foil.

10. Bake for 30-35 minutes until peppers are tender.

11. Remove foil, sprinkle with shredded cheddar cheese if using, and bake for an additional 5 minutes until cheese is melted.

12. Garnish with fresh cilantro before serving.

Nutrition Information (per serving):

- Calories: 280
- Protein: 10g
- Carbohydrates: 35g
- Fat: 10g
- Fiber: 8g
- Sugar: 8g
- Portion size: 1 stuffed pepper

## Mushroom and Spinach Stuffed Portobello

Ingredients:

- Portobello mushrooms
- Baby spinach
- Garlic, minced
- Olive oil
- Cream cheese (or goat cheese for tangy flavor)
- Parmesan cheese, grated
- Italian seasoning

- Salt and pepper

Instructions:

1. Preheat oven to 375°F (190°C).
2. Clean mushrooms and remove stems.
3. In a skillet, heat olive oil over medium heat.
4. Sauté minced garlic until fragrant, then add baby spinach and cook until wilted.
5. Remove from heat and stir in cream cheese (or goat cheese), Parmesan cheese, Italian seasoning, salt, and pepper.
6. Spoon spinach mixture into each mushroom cap.
7. Place stuffed mushrooms on a baking sheet lined with parchment paper.
8. Bake for 20-25 minutes until mushrooms are tender and filling is heated through.
9. Serve hot, garnished with additional Parmesan cheese if desired.

Nutrition Information (per serving):

- Calories: 200
- Protein: 12g
- Carbohydrates: 10g
- Fat: 15g
- Fiber: 5g

- Sugar: 3g
- Portion size: 1 stuffed mushroom

## Greek Salad with Tofu

Ingredients:
- Firm tofu, cubed
- Cucumber, diced
- Cherry tomatoes, halved
- Red onion, thinly sliced
- Kalamata olives, pitted
- Feta cheese, crumbled (optional)
- Fresh parsley, chopped
- Olive oil
- Red wine vinegar
- Dried oregano
- Salt and pepper

Instructions:
1. Heat olive oil in a skillet over medium-high heat.
2. Add cubed tofu and cook until golden brown on all sides.
3. In a large bowl, combine cucumber, cherry tomatoes, red onion, Kalamata olives, and parsley.

4.  In a small bowl, whisk together olive oil, red wine vinegar, dried oregano, salt, and pepper to make the dressing.

5.  Add cooked tofu and feta cheese to the salad ingredients.

6.  Pour the dressing over the salad and toss gently to combine.

7.  Adjust seasoning if needed before serving.

Nutrition Information (per serving):

- Calories: 250
- Protein: 15g
- Carbohydrates: 15g
- Fat: 15g
- Fiber: 5g
- Sugar: 5g
- Portion size: 1 cup

## Roasted Veggie Buddha Bowl

Ingredients:

- Sweet potatoes, cubed
- Brussels sprouts, halved
- Chickpeas (canned, drained and rinsed)
- Red onion, sliced
- Olive oil
- Garlic powder

- Paprika
- Tahini sauce (homemade or store-bought)
- Fresh parsley, chopped
- Lemon wedges

Instructions:

1. Preheat oven to 400°F (200°C).
2. Toss sweet potatoes, Brussels sprouts, chickpeas, and red onion with olive oil, garlic powder, and paprika on a baking sheet.
3. Roast in the oven for 30-35 minutes until vegetables are tender and slightly caramelized.
4. Divide roasted vegetables and chickpeas into serving bowls.
5. Drizzle with tahini sauce and garnish with fresh parsley.
6. Serve with lemon wedges for squeezing over the bowl.

Nutrition Information (per serving):

- Calories: 300
- Protein: 12g
- Carbohydrates: 35g
- Fat: 12g
- Fiber: 10g
- Sugar: 8g
- Portion size: 1 bowl

## Low Carb Veggie Tacos

Ingredients:

- Low carb tortillas (or lettuce leaves for wrapping)
- Cauliflower florets
- Bell peppers, sliced
- Red cabbage, shredded
- Avocado, sliced
- Cilantro, chopped
- Lime wedges
- Olive oil
- Cumin
- Chili powder
- Salt and pepper

Instructions:

1. Preheat oven to 400°F (200°C).
2. Toss cauliflower florets and bell peppers with olive oil, cumin, chili powder, salt, and pepper on a baking sheet.
3. Roast in the oven for 20-25 minutes until vegetables are tender and slightly charred.
4. Heat low carb tortillas in a dry skillet or microwave according to package instructions.
5. Assemble tacos with roasted vegetables, shredded red cabbage, avocado slices, and chopped cilantro.

6.  Serve with lime wedges for squeezing over the tacos.

Nutrition Information (per serving):

- Calories: 220

- Protein: 8g

- Carbohydrates: 20g

- Fat: 12g

- Fiber: 8g

- Sugar: 5g

- Portion size: 2 tacos

## Cauliflower Pizza with Veggie Toppings

Ingredients:

- Cauliflower crust (store-bought or homemade)

- Low carb marinara sauce

- Mozzarella cheese, shredded

- Assorted vegetables (bell peppers, mushrooms, onions, spinach)

- Olive oil

- Italian seasoning

- Salt and pepper

Instructions:

1.  Preheat oven according to cauliflower crust package instructions or recipe guidelines.
2.  Prepare cauliflower crust as directed, ensuring it is cooked and slightly crispy.
3.  Spread a thin layer of low carb marinara sauce over the crust.
4.  Sprinkle shredded mozzarella cheese evenly over the sauce.
5.  Arrange sliced vegetables on top of the cheese.
6.  Drizzle with olive oil and sprinkle with Italian seasoning, salt, and pepper.
7.  Bake pizza in the oven until cheese is melted and vegetables are cooked to your liking.
8.  Remove from oven and let cool slightly before slicing and serving.

Nutrition Information (per serving):

- Calories: 250
- Protein: 12g
- Carbohydrates: 20g
- Fat: 15g
- Fiber: 8g
- Sugar: 5g
- Portion size: 1/4 of pizza

# Cucumber and Avocado Gazpacho

Ingredients:

- Cucumbers, peeled and chopped
- Avocado, peeled and pitted
- Greek yogurt (or coconut yogurt for vegan option)
- Fresh cilantro, chopped
- Lime juice
- Garlic, minced
- Jalapeño, seeded and chopped (optional)
- Vegetable broth
- Salt and pepper

Instructions:

1. In a blender, combine chopped cucumbers, avocado, Greek yogurt, cilantro, lime juice, minced garlic, and jalapeño.
2. Blend until smooth, adding vegetable broth as needed to achieve desired consistency.
3. Season with salt and pepper to taste.
4. Chill gazpacho in the refrigerator for at least 1 hour before serving.
5. Stir well before serving and garnish with additional chopped cilantro if desired.

Nutrition Information (per serving):

- Calories: 180
- Protein: 6g
- Carbohydrates: 15g
- Fat: 10g
- Fiber: 8g
- Sugar: 5g
- Portion size: 1 cup

# Chapter 4: Dinner Recipes

In this chapter, you'll discover a variety of flavorful dinner recipes designed for those following a low-carb vegetarian diet, especially beneficial for managing Type 2 diabetes. Each recipe features nutritious ingredients that are both satisfying and delicious, ensuring you can enjoy a wholesome meal without compromising on taste or health goals.

## Eggplant Lasagna

Ingredients:

- 2 medium eggplants, thinly sliced
- 2 cups marinara sauce
- 1 cup ricotta cheese
- 1 cup shredded mozzarella cheese
- 1/4 cup grated Parmesan cheese
- Fresh basil leaves for garnish

Instructions:

1. Preheat oven to 375°F (190°C).
2. Layer marinara sauce, eggplant slices, ricotta cheese, and mozzarella cheese in a baking dish.
3. Repeat layers, ending with mozzarella and Parmesan on top.

4. Bake for 30 minutes until bubbly and golden.

5. Garnish with fresh basil leaves before serving.

Nutrition Information per serving:

- Calories: 320

- Protein: 15g

- Carbohydrates: 20g

- Fat: 20g

- Fiber: 8g

- Sugar: 12g

- Portion size: 1/6 of the lasagna

## Cauliflower Crust Pizza

Ingredients:

- 1 medium cauliflower, grated

- 1 cup shredded mozzarella cheese

- 1 egg

- 1/2 tsp dried oregano

- 1/2 tsp garlic powder

- 1/4 cup marinara sauce

- Assorted vegetable toppings (bell peppers, onions, mushrooms)

Instructions:

1.  Preheat oven to 400°F (200°C).

2.  Mix cauliflower, mozzarella, egg, oregano, and garlic powder in a bowl.

3.  Press mixture into a pizza crust shape on a baking sheet lined with parchment paper.

4.  Bake for 20 minutes until golden brown.

5.  Spread marinara sauce and add vegetable toppings.

6.  Bake for an additional 10 minutes until cheese is melted.

Nutrition Information per serving:

- Calories: 250
- Protein: 14g
- Carbohydrates: 12g
- Fat: 15g
- Fiber: 5g
- Sugar: 5g
- Portion size: 1/4 of the pizza

## Stuffed Zucchini Boats

Ingredients:

- 4 medium zucchinis, halved lengthwise
- 1 cup quinoa, cooked

- 1 cup cherry tomatoes, halved
- 1/2 cup crumbled feta cheese
- 1/4 cup chopped fresh basil
- Salt and pepper to taste

Instructions:

1. Preheat oven to 375°F (190°C).
2. Scoop out zucchini flesh, leaving a 1/4-inch shell.
3. Mix quinoa, tomatoes, feta, basil, salt, and pepper in a bowl.
4. Stuff zucchini halves with quinoa mixture.
5. Bake for 25-30 minutes until zucchini is tender.

Nutrition Information per serving:

- Calories: 280
- Protein: 12g
- Carbohydrates: 30g
- Fat: 12g
- Fiber: 6g
- Sugar: 8g
- Portion size: 2 zucchini halves

# Keto Veggie Stir-Fry with Tofu

Ingredients:

- 1 block firm tofu, drained and cubed
- 2 cups mixed vegetables (broccoli, bell peppers, snap peas)
- 2 tbsp soy sauce (low sodium)
- 1 tbsp sesame oil
- 2 cloves garlic, minced
- 1 tsp ginger, grated
- Sesame seeds for garnish

Instructions:

1. Heat sesame oil in a large pan over medium-high heat.
2. Add tofu cubes and stir-fry until golden brown, about 5-7 minutes.
3. Add garlic and ginger, cook for 1 minute until fragrant.
4. Add mixed vegetables and soy sauce, stir-fry for another 3-4 minutes until vegetables are tender-crisp.
5. Garnish with sesame seeds before serving.

Nutrition Information per serving:

- Calories: 280
- Protein: 18g
- Carbohydrates: 14g
- Fat: 16g

- Fiber: 5g

- Sugar: 6g

- Portion size: 1/4 of the stir-fry

## Creamy Spinach and Mushroom Casserole

Ingredients:

- 2 cups spinach, chopped

- 2 cups mushrooms, sliced

- 1 cup heavy cream

- 1/2 cup grated Parmesan cheese

- 2 cloves garlic, minced

- Salt and pepper to taste

Instructions:

1. Preheat oven to 375°F (190°C).

2. In a skillet, sauté mushrooms and garlic until mushrooms are golden.

3. Add spinach and cook until wilted.

4. Stir in heavy cream, Parmesan cheese, salt, and pepper.

5. Transfer mixture to a baking dish and bake for 20-25 minutes until bubbly and golden.

Nutrition Information per serving:

- Calories: 320
- Protein: 12g
- Carbohydrates: 8g
- Fat: 28g
- Fiber: 2g
- Sugar: 3g
- Portion size: 1/4 of the casserole

# Grilled Portobello Mushrooms with Avocado Salsa

Ingredients:

- 4 large portobello mushrooms
- 2 avocados, diced
- 1 tomato, diced
- 1/4 cup red onion, finely chopped
- 2 tbsp cilantro, chopped
- Juice of 1 lime
- Salt and pepper to taste

Instructions:

1. Preheat grill or grill pan over medium-high heat.

2.  Remove stems from portobello mushrooms and brush with olive oil.

3.  Grill mushrooms for 5-7 minutes on each side until tender.

4.  In a bowl, mix diced avocado, tomato, red onion, cilantro, lime juice, salt, and pepper.

5.  Spoon avocado salsa over grilled mushrooms before serving.

Nutrition Information per serving:

- Calories: 240
- Protein: 6g
- Carbohydrates: 18g
- Fat: 18g
- Fiber: 10g
- Sugar: 4g
- Portion size: 1 mushroom with salsa

## Ratatouille

Ingredients:

- 1 eggplant, diced
- 2 zucchinis, diced
- 1 bell pepper, diced
- 1 onion, diced
- 2 cloves garlic, minced

- 2 cups tomato sauce
- 1 tsp dried thyme
- 1 tsp dried oregano
- Salt and pepper to taste
- Fresh basil leaves for garnish

Instructions:

1. Heat olive oil in a large skillet over medium heat.
2. Add onion and garlic, sauté until softened.
3. Add eggplant, zucchini, and bell pepper, cook for 5-7 minutes until vegetables are slightly tender.
4. Stir in tomato sauce, thyme, oregano, salt, and pepper.
5. Simmer for 15-20 minutes until vegetables are cooked through.
6. Garnish with fresh basil leaves before serving.

Nutrition Information per serving:

- Calories: 180
- Protein: 5g
- Carbohydrates: 25g
- Fat: 7g
- Fiber: 8g
- Sugar: 12g
- Portion size: 1/4 of the ratatouille

# Spaghetti Squash Alfredo

Ingredients:

- 1 medium spaghetti squash
- 1 cup Alfredo sauce (low carb)
- 1 cup spinach, chopped
- 1/4 cup grated Parmesan cheese
- Salt and pepper to taste

Instructions:

1. Preheat oven to 400°F (200°C).
2. Cut spaghetti squash in half lengthwise and scoop out seeds.
3. Place squash halves cut-side down on a baking sheet lined with parchment paper.
4. Bake for 30-40 minutes until tender.
5. Scrape squash flesh with a fork to create "spaghetti" strands.
6. In a saucepan, heat Alfredo sauce and spinach until spinach is wilted.
7. Toss spaghetti squash with Alfredo sauce mixture.
8. Stir in Parmesan cheese, salt, and pepper before serving.

Nutrition Information per serving:

- Calories: 280
- Protein: 10g
- Carbohydrates: 20g

- Fat: 18g
- Fiber: 5g
- Sugar: 8g
- Portion size: 1/2 of the spaghetti squash

## Thai Coconut Curry with Vegetables

Ingredients:

- 1 can coconut milk
- 2 cups mixed vegetables (bell peppers, broccoli, carrots)
- 1 block tofu, cubed
- 2 tbsp Thai red curry paste
- 1 tbsp soy sauce (low sodium)
- Fresh cilantro for garnish

Instructions:

1. In a large pan, heat coconut milk over medium heat.
2. Stir in Thai red curry paste and soy sauce until well combined.
3. Add mixed vegetables and tofu cubes, simmer for 10-15 minutes until vegetables are tender.
4. Garnish with fresh cilantro before serving.

Nutrition Information per serving:

- Calories: 320
- Protein: 15g
- Carbohydrates: 18g
- Fat: 22g
- Fiber: 5g
- Sugar: 8g
- Portion size: 1/4 of the curry

## Cauliflower Mac and Cheese

Ingredients:

- 1 medium head cauliflower, chopped into florets
- 1 cup shredded cheddar cheese
- 1/2 cup heavy cream
- 1/4 cup grated Parmesan cheese
- 1/2 tsp garlic powder
- Salt and pepper to taste
- Fresh parsley for garnish

Instructions:

1. Preheat oven to 375°F (190°C).
2. Steam cauliflower florets until tender, about 5-7 minutes.
3. In a saucepan, heat heavy cream over medium heat.

4.  Stir in cheddar cheese, Parmesan cheese, garlic powder, salt, and pepper until smooth and creamy.

5.  Add steamed cauliflower to the cheese sauce, mix well.

6.  Transfer mixture to a baking dish and bake for 15-20 minutes until bubbly and golden.

7.  Garnish with fresh parsley before serving.

Nutrition Information per serving:

- Calories: 280
- Protein: 12g
- Carbohydrates: 10g
- Fat: 20g
- Fiber: 4g
- Sugar: 5g
- Portion size: 1/4 of the cauliflower mac and cheese

## Grilled Asparagus with Lemon-Garlic Sauce

Ingredients:

- 1 bunch asparagus, trimmed
- 2 tbsp olive oil
- 2 cloves garlic, minced
- Zest and juice of 1 lemon

- Salt and pepper to taste

Instructions:

1. Preheat grill or grill pan over medium-high heat.
2. Toss asparagus with olive oil, salt, and pepper.
3. Grill asparagus for 3-4 minutes per side until tender and charred.
4. In a small bowl, mix minced garlic, lemon zest, and lemon juice.
5. Drizzle lemon-garlic sauce over grilled asparagus before serving.

Nutrition Information per serving:

- Calories: 120
- Protein: 4g
- Carbohydrates: 8g
- Fat: 9g
- Fiber: 4g
- Sugar: 2g
- Portion size: 1/2 of the grilled asparagus

# Brussels Sprouts with Walnuts and Balsamic Reduction

Ingredients:

- 1 lb Brussels sprouts, trimmed and halved
- 1/2 cup walnuts, chopped
- 2 tbsp olive oil
- 2 tbsp balsamic vinegar
- Salt and pepper to taste

Instructions:

1. Preheat oven to 400°F (200°C).
2. Toss Brussels sprouts with olive oil, salt, and pepper.
3. Roast Brussels sprouts for 20-25 minutes until tender and caramelized.
4. In a small saucepan, simmer balsamic vinegar until reduced by half.
5. Stir in walnuts and roasted Brussels sprouts, toss to combine.
6. Serve warm.

Nutrition Information per serving:

- Calories: 180
- Protein: 6g
- Carbohydrates: 12g
- Fat: 14g

- Fiber: 4g

- Sugar: 4g

- Portion size: 1/4 of the Brussels sprouts


## Stuffed Acorn Squash

Ingredients:

- 2 acorn squashes, halved and seeded

- 1 cup quinoa, cooked

- 1 cup kale, chopped

- 1/2 cup dried cranberries

- 1/4 cup pecans, chopped

- 1/4 cup feta cheese, crumbled

- 1 tbsp olive oil

- Salt and pepper to taste

Instructions:

1. Preheat oven to 400°F (200°C).

2. Brush acorn squash halves with olive oil, season with salt and pepper.

3. Place squash halves cut-side down on a baking sheet lined with parchment paper.

4. Bake for 30-35 minutes until squash is tender.

5. In a bowl, mix cooked quinoa, kale, dried cranberries, pecans, and feta cheese.

6. Stuff squash halves with quinoa mixture.

7. Bake for an additional 10 minutes until filling is heated through.

Nutrition Information per serving:

- Calories: 320
- Protein: 10g
- Carbohydrates: 45g
- Fat: 12g
- Fiber: 8g
- Sugar: 10g
- Portion size: 1/2 of the stuffed acorn squash

## Broccoli Cheddar Casserole

Ingredients:

- 4 cups broccoli florets
- 1 cup shredded cheddar cheese
- 1/2 cup heavy cream
- 2 tbsp cream cheese
- 1/4 cup grated Parmesan cheese
- 1/2 tsp garlic powder

- Salt and pepper to taste

Instructions:

1. Preheat oven to 375°F (190°C).
2. Steam broccoli florets until tender, about 5-7 minutes.
3. In a saucepan, heat heavy cream over medium heat.
4. Stir in cream cheese, cheddar cheese, Parmesan cheese, garlic powder, salt, and pepper until smooth and creamy.
5. Add steamed broccoli to the cheese sauce, mix well.
6. Transfer mixture to a baking dish and bake for 15-20 minutes until bubbly and golden.

Nutrition Information per serving:

- Calories: 280
- Protein: 12g
- Carbohydrates: 10g
- Fat: 20g
- Fiber: 4g
- Sugar: 5g
- Portion size: 1/4 of the casserole

# Roasted Vegetable Medley

Ingredients:

- 2 cups mixed vegetables (bell peppers, carrots, onions, zucchini)
- 2 tbsp olive oil
- 1 tsp dried Italian seasoning
- Salt and pepper to taste

Instructions:

1. Preheat oven to 400°F (200°C).
2. Cut vegetables into bite-sized pieces and place on a baking sheet.
3. Drizzle olive oil over vegetables, sprinkle with Italian seasoning, salt, and pepper.
4. Toss vegetables to coat evenly with oil and seasonings.
5. Roast in the oven for 20-25 minutes, stirring halfway through, until vegetables are tender and slightly caramelized.

Nutrition Information per serving:

- Calories: 150
- Protein: 3g
- Carbohydrates: 12g
- Fat: 10g
- Fiber: 4g

- Sugar: 6g

- Portion size: 1/2 cup of the roasted vegetable medley

# Chapter 5: Snacks and Appetizers

In between meals or as a prelude to dinner, these snacks and appetizers are designed to satisfy cravings while keeping your carbohydrate intake in check. From crunchy veggies with creamy dips to savory stuffed bites, each recipe offers a delicious option for any occasion.

## Guacamole with Cucumber Slices

Ingredients:

- 2 ripe avocados
- 1 small tomato, diced
- 1/4 cup red onion, finely chopped
- 1 jalapeño, seeded and minced (optional)
- Juice of 1 lime
- Salt and pepper to taste
- Fresh cilantro, chopped
- Cucumber slices, for serving

Instructions:

1. In a bowl, mash the avocados with a fork until smooth.
2. Stir in the diced tomato, red onion, jalapeño (if using), lime juice, salt, and pepper.

3. Garnish with chopped cilantro.

4. Serve with cucumber slices.

Nutrition Information (per serving):

- Calories: 120

- Protein: 2g

- Carbohydrates: 8g

- Fat: 10g

- Fiber: 6g

- Sugar: 1g

- Portion Size: 1/4 cup guacamole with 5 cucumber slices

## Stuffed Mini Bell Peppers

Ingredients:

- 12 mini bell peppers, halved and seeded

- 1 cup cream cheese, softened

- 1/2 cup shredded cheddar cheese

- 1/4 cup chopped fresh chives

- Salt and pepper to taste

Instructions:

1. In a bowl, mix together the cream cheese, cheddar cheese, chives, salt, and pepper until well combined.

2. Spoon the mixture into each mini bell pepper half.

3. Arrange on a serving platter and serve chilled or at room temperature.

Nutrition Information (per serving, 2 halves):

- Calories: 120
- Protein: 4g
- Carbohydrates: 6g
- Fat: 9g
- Fiber: 2g
- Sugar: 3g
- Portion Size: 2 stuffed pepper halves

## Kale Chips

Ingredients:

- 1 bunch kale, washed and dried
- 1-2 tablespoons olive oil
- Salt to taste

Instructions:

1. Preheat oven to 350°F (175°C).

2. Remove the kale leaves from the stems and tear into bite-sized pieces.

3.  Drizzle with olive oil and massage into the kale leaves.

4.  Spread out on a baking sheet in a single layer.

5.  Sprinkle with salt.

6.  Bake for 10-15 minutes until crispy, checking frequently to prevent burning.

Nutrition Information (per serving):

- Calories: 50
- Protein: 2g
- Carbohydrates: 5g
- Fat: 3g
- Fiber: 1g
- Sugar: 0g
- Portion Size: 1 cup kale chips

## Roasted Chickpeas

Ingredients:

- 1 can (15 oz) chickpeas, drained and rinsed
- 1 tablespoon olive oil
- 1 teaspoon ground cumin
- 1/2 teaspoon paprika
- Salt to taste

Instructions:

1.  Preheat oven to 400°F (200°C).
2.  Pat chickpeas dry with a paper towel.
3.  In a bowl, toss chickpeas with olive oil, cumin, paprika, and salt.
4.  Spread out on a baking sheet in a single layer.
5.  Bake for 20-25 minutes, shaking the pan halfway through, until golden and crispy.

Nutrition Information (per serving):

- Calories: 150
- Protein: 6g
- Carbohydrates: 22g
- Fat: 5g
- Fiber: 6g
- Sugar: 4g
- Portion Size: 1/2 cup roasted chickpeas

## Veggie Sticks with Hummus

Ingredients:

- Assorted vegetables (carrots, celery, bell peppers, cucumber), cut into sticks
- Store-bought or homemade hummus

Instructions:

1. Arrange vegetable sticks on a plate.
2. Serve with hummus for dipping.

Nutrition Information (per serving):

- Calories: 80
- Protein: 4g
- Carbohydrates: 12g
- Fat: 3g
- Fiber: 5g
- Sugar: 5g
- Portion Size: 1 cup vegetable sticks with 2 tablespoons hummus

## Almond Butter and Celery Sticks

Ingredients:

- Celery stalks, washed and cut into sticks
- Almond butter

Instructions:

1. Spread almond butter into the groove of each celery stick.
2. Arrange on a plate and serve.

Nutrition Information (per serving):

- Calories: 100
- Protein: 3g
- Carbohydrates: 6g
- Fat: 8g
- Fiber: 3g
- Sugar: 2g
- Portion Size: 2 celery sticks with 1 tablespoon almond butter

## Zucchini Chips

Ingredients:

- 2 medium zucchinis, thinly sliced
- 1 tablespoon olive oil
- Salt and pepper to taste

Instructions:

1. Preheat oven to 225°F (110°C).
2. Toss zucchini slices with olive oil, salt, and pepper.
3. Arrange in a single layer on a baking sheet lined with parchment paper.
4. Bake for 2-3 hours until crispy, flipping halfway through.

Nutrition Information (per serving):

- Calories: 60
- Protein: 2g
- Carbohydrates: 6g
- Fat: 4g
- Fiber: 2g
- Sugar: 3g
- Portion Size: 1 cup zucchini chips

## Cauliflower Buffalo Bites

Ingredients:

- 1 head cauliflower, cut into florets
- 1/2 cup buffalo sauce
- 1 tablespoon olive oil
- Salt and pepper to taste

Instructions:

1. Preheat oven to 450°F (230°C).
2. Toss cauliflower florets with olive oil, salt, and pepper.
3. Arrange on a baking sheet and bake for 20 minutes, flipping halfway through.
4. Remove from oven and toss with buffalo sauce.
5. Return to oven for an additional 10 minutes until crispy.

Nutrition Information (per serving):

- Calories: 70
- Protein: 3g
- Carbohydrates: 8g
- Fat: 3g
- Fiber: 3g
- Sugar: 3g
- Portion Size: 1 cup cauliflower buffalo bites

## Edamame with Sea Salt

Ingredients:

- 2 cups edamame (fresh or frozen)
- Sea salt to taste

Instructions:

1. Boil or steam edamame according to package instructions.
2. Drain and sprinkle with sea salt.
3. Serve warm or chilled.

Nutrition Information (per serving):

- Calories: 150
- Protein: 14g
- Carbohydrates: 11g

- Fat: 6g

- Fiber: 9g

- Sugar: 3g

- Portion Size: 1 cup edamame

## Cheese and Olive Platter

Ingredients:

- Assorted cheeses (cheddar, brie, goat cheese)

- Assorted olives (green, Kalamata)

- Crackers (optional)

Instructions:

1. Arrange cheeses and olives on a platter.

2. Serve with crackers if desired.

Nutrition Information (per serving):

- Calories: 200

- Protein: 10g

- Carbohydrates: 5g

- Fat: 15g

- Fiber: 2g

- Sugar: 1g

- Portion Size: 1 ounce cheese with 1/4 cup olives

# Spinach and Artichoke Dip

Ingredients:

- 1 cup frozen spinach, thawed and drained
- 1 can (14 oz) artichoke hearts, drained and chopped
- 1 cup plain Greek yogurt
- 1/2 cup shredded mozzarella cheese
- 1/4 cup grated Parmesan cheese
- 1 clove garlic, minced
- Salt and pepper to taste

Instructions:

1. Preheat oven to 375°F (190°C).
2. In a bowl, combine spinach, artichoke hearts, Greek yogurt, mozzarella cheese, Parmesan cheese, garlic, salt, and pepper.
3. Transfer mixture to a baking dish.
4. Bake for 20-25 minutes until bubbly and golden brown on top.
5. Serve warm with vegetable sticks or whole grain crackers.

Nutrition Information (per serving):

- Calories: 120
- Protein: 10g
- Carbohydrates: 7g
- Fat: 6g

- Fiber: 3g

- Sugar: 2g

- Portion Size: 1/4 cup dip

## Mini Caprese Skewers

Ingredients:

- Cherry tomatoes

- Fresh basil leaves

- Mozzarella balls (bocconcini)

- Balsamic glaze (optional)

Instructions:

1. Thread cherry tomatoes, basil leaves, and mozzarella balls onto small skewers.

2. Arrange on a serving platter.

3. Drizzle with balsamic glaze if desired.

4. Serve chilled.

Nutrition Information (per serving):

- Calories: 100

- Protein: 7g

- Carbohydrates: 3g

- Fat: 6g

- Fiber: 1g

- Sugar: 2g

- Portion Size: 4 skewers

## Cucumber Roll-Ups with Avocado

Ingredients:

- 1 cucumber

- 1 avocado, mashed

- 1/4 cup shredded carrots

- 1/4 cup baby spinach leaves

Instructions:

1. Slice cucumber lengthwise into thin strips using a vegetable peeler or mandoline.

2. Spread mashed avocado onto each cucumber strip.

3. Top with shredded carrots and spinach leaves.

4. Roll up each cucumber strip and secure with a toothpick if needed.

5. Serve chilled.

Nutrition Information (per serving):

- Calories: 90

- Protein: 2g

- Carbohydrates: 7g

- Fat: 6g

- Fiber: 4g

- Sugar: 2g

- Portion Size: 4 roll-ups

## Broccoli Tots

Ingredients:

- 2 cups broccoli florets, steamed and finely chopped

- 1/2 cup shredded cheddar cheese

- 1/4 cup almond flour

- 1 egg

- 1/2 teaspoon garlic powder

- Salt and pepper to taste

Instructions:

1. Preheat oven to 400°F (200°C). Line a baking sheet with parchment paper.

2. In a bowl, combine chopped broccoli, cheddar cheese, almond flour, egg, garlic powder, salt, and pepper.

3. Shape mixture into tots and place on the baking sheet.

4. Bake for 20-25 minutes until golden and crispy.

5. Serve hot with a dipping sauce of your choice.

Nutrition Information (per serving):

- Calories: 120
- Protein: 7g
- Carbohydrates: 6g
- Fat: 8g
- Fiber: 3g
- Sugar: 2g
- Portion Size: 5 tots

## Stuffed Mushrooms

Ingredients:

- 12 large mushrooms, stems removed and finely chopped
- 1/2 cup cream cheese, softened
- 1/4 cup grated Parmesan cheese
- 1/4 cup chopped fresh parsley
- 2 cloves garlic, minced
- Salt and pepper to taste

Instructions:

1. Preheat oven to 375°F (190°C). Line a baking sheet with parchment paper.
2. In a bowl, mix together chopped mushroom stems, cream cheese, Parmesan cheese, parsley, garlic, salt, and pepper.

3. Spoon mixture into each mushroom cap, filling generously.

4. Place stuffed mushrooms on the baking sheet.

5. Bake for 15-20 minutes until mushrooms are tender and filling is golden brown.

6. Serve warm.

Nutrition Information (per serving, 2 mushrooms):

- Calories: 100
- Protein: 6g
- Carbohydrates: 4g
- Fat: 7g
- Fiber: 1g
- Sugar: 2g
- Portion Size: 2 stuffed mushrooms

# Chapter 6: Desserts

Welcome to the sweet finale of your low carb vegetarian journey for managing Type 2 Diabetes! Indulging in desserts while keeping your health in check is absolutely possible with these delicious recipes. Each dessert is crafted to satisfy your cravings without compromising your dietary goals. Enjoy experimenting with these treats and savor guilt-free delights that support your well-being.

## Avocado Chocolate Mousse

Ingredients:

- 2 ripe avocados
- 1/4 cup unsweetened cocoa powder
- 1/4 cup almond milk
- 1/4 cup keto-friendly sweetener (like erythritol or stevia)
- 1 tsp vanilla extract

Instructions:

1. Blend all ingredients in a food processor until smooth.
2. Chill in the refrigerator for at least 1 hour before serving.

Nutrition Information (per serving):

- Calories: 180

- Protein: 3g
- Carbohydrates: 12g
- Fat: 15g
- Fiber: 7g
- Sugar: 1g
- Portion size: 1/2 cup

## Almond Flour Brownies

Ingredients:

- 1 cup almond flour
- 1/4 cup unsweetened cocoa powder
- 1/2 cup keto-friendly sweetener
- 1/4 cup melted butter
- 2 large eggs
- 1 tsp vanilla extract
- 1/4 tsp salt

Instructions:

1. Preheat oven to 350°F (175°C). Grease a baking dish.
2. Mix almond flour, cocoa powder, sweetener, and salt in a bowl.
3. Stir in melted butter, eggs, and vanilla extract until well combined.

4. Pour batter into the prepared dish and bake for 20-25
   minutes.

5. Let cool before cutting into squares.

Nutrition Information (per serving):

- Calories: 120
- Protein: 4g
- Carbohydrates: 6g
- Fat: 9g
- Fiber: 2g
- Sugar: 1g
- Portion size: 1 brownie

## Keto Cheesecake Bites

Ingredients:

- 8 oz cream cheese, softened
- 1/4 cup keto-friendly sweetener
- 1 tsp vanilla extract
- 1 large egg
- 1/4 cup almond flour

Instructions:

1. Preheat oven to 325°F (160°C). Line a mini muffin tin with paper liners.
2. Beat cream cheese, sweetener, and vanilla extract until smooth.
3. Add egg and beat until combined.
4. Spoon batter into muffin tin, filling each about 2/3 full.
5. Sprinkle almond flour on top of each cheesecake bite.
6. Bake for 15-18 minutes until set.
7. Cool completely before serving.

Nutrition Information (per serving - 2 cheesecake bites):

- Calories: 180
- Protein: 4g
- Carbohydrates: 3g
- Fat: 17g
- Fiber: 1g
- Sugar: 2g
- Portion size: 2 cheesecake bites

## Chia Seed Pudding

Ingredients:

- 1/4 cup chia seeds

- 1 cup unsweetened almond milk
- 1 tbsp keto-friendly sweetener (optional)
- 1/2 tsp vanilla extract
- Berries or nuts for topping (optional)

Instructions:

1. In a bowl, mix chia seeds, almond milk, sweetener (if using), and vanilla extract.
2. Stir well to combine and let sit for 10 minutes.
3. Stir again to break up any clumps of chia seeds.
4. Cover and refrigerate for at least 2 hours or overnight.
5. Serve chilled with berries or nuts on top, if desired.

Nutrition Information (per serving):

- Calories: 120
- Protein: 4g
- Carbohydrates: 10g
- Fat: 7g
- Fiber: 8g
- Sugar: 0g
- Portion size: 1/2 cup

# Coconut Flour Cookies

Ingredients:

- 1/2 cup coconut flour
- 1/4 cup keto-friendly sweetener
- 1/4 cup melted coconut oil
- 2 large eggs
- 1/2 tsp vanilla extract
- Pinch of salt

Instructions:

1. Preheat oven to 350°F (175°C). Line a baking sheet with parchment paper.
2. In a bowl, mix coconut flour, sweetener, and salt.
3. Add melted coconut oil, eggs, and vanilla extract. Mix until dough forms.
4. Roll dough into small balls and place on the baking sheet.
5. Flatten each ball with a fork.
6. Bake for 12-15 minutes until edges are golden brown.
7. Let cool on the baking sheet before transferring to a wire rack.

Nutrition Information (per serving - 2 cookies):

- Calories: 120
- Protein: 3g

- Carbohydrates: 7g

- Fat: 9g

- Fiber: 3g

- Sugar: 1g

- Portion size: 2 cookies

## Berry Crumble

Ingredients:

- 2 cups mixed berries (such as strawberries, blueberries, raspberries)
- 1/2 cup almond flour
- 1/4 cup keto-friendly sweetener
- 1/4 cup melted butter
- 1/2 tsp cinnamon

Instructions:

1. Preheat oven to 350°F (175°C). Grease a baking dish.
2. Spread berries evenly in the bottom of the dish.
3. In a bowl, combine almond flour, sweetener, melted butter, and cinnamon until crumbly.
4. Sprinkle crumble mixture over the berries.
5. Bake for 25-30 minutes until topping is golden brown and berries are bubbly.

6. Let cool slightly before serving.

Nutrition Information (per serving):

- Calories: 150

- Protein: 3g

- Carbohydrates: 10g

- Fat: 12g

- Fiber: 4g

- Sugar: 5g

- Portion size: 1/2 cup

## Lemon Coconut Balls

Ingredients:

- 1 cup shredded unsweetened coconut

- 1/4 cup almond flour

- 2 tbsp keto-friendly sweetener

- Zest of 1 lemon

- 2 tbsp lemon juice

- 2 tbsp melted coconut oil

Instructions:

1. In a food processor, blend shredded coconut until finely chopped.

2.  Add almond flour, sweetener, lemon zest, lemon juice, and melted coconut oil. Pulse until mixture sticks together.

3.  Roll mixture into balls about 1 inch in diameter.

4.  Optional: Roll balls in additional shredded coconut or almond flour for coating.

5.  Refrigerate for at least 30 minutes before serving.

Nutrition Information (per serving - 2 balls):

- Calories: 120
- Protein: 2g
- Carbohydrates: 5g
- Fat: 10g
- Fiber: 3g
- Sugar: 2g
- Portion size: 2 balls

## Chocolate Zucchini Bread

Ingredients:

- 1 cup shredded zucchini (excess water squeezed out)
- 1 cup almond flour
- 1/4 cup cocoa powder
- 1/4 cup keto-friendly sweetener
- 1/4 cup melted coconut oil

- 2 large eggs
- 1 tsp vanilla extract
- 1/2 tsp baking soda
- Pinch of salt

Instructions:

1. Preheat oven to 350°F (175°C). Grease a loaf pan.
2. In a bowl, mix almond flour, cocoa powder, sweetener, baking soda, and salt.
3. In another bowl, whisk together melted coconut oil, eggs, and vanilla extract.
4. Combine wet and dry ingredients, then fold in shredded zucchini until evenly distributed.
5. Pour batter into the loaf pan and spread evenly.
6. Bake for 45-50 minutes or until a toothpick inserted into the center comes out clean.
7. Let cool in the pan for 10 minutes before transferring to a wire rack to cool completely.

Nutrition Information (per serving - 1 slice):

- Calories: 150
- Protein: 5g
- Carbohydrates: 7g
- Fat: 12g

- Fiber: 3g

- Sugar: 2g

- Portion size: 1 slice

## Pumpkin Spice Muffins

Ingredients:

- 1 cup almond flour

- 1/4 cup coconut flour

- 1/4 cup keto-friendly sweetener

- 1 tsp baking powder

- 1/2 tsp baking soda

- 1/2 tsp cinnamon

- 1/4 tsp nutmeg

- 1/4 tsp cloves

- 1/2 cup pumpkin puree

- 1/4 cup melted coconut oil

- 2 large eggs

- 1 tsp vanilla extract

Instructions:

1. Preheat oven to 350°F (175°C). Line a muffin tin with paper liners.

2. In a bowl, whisk together almond flour, coconut flour, sweetener, baking powder, baking soda, cinnamon, nutmeg, and cloves.

3. In another bowl, mix pumpkin puree, melted coconut oil, eggs, and vanilla extract until smooth.

4. Combine wet and dry ingredients until well incorporated.

5. Spoon batter into muffin tin, filling each about 3/4 full.

6. Bake for 20-25 minutes or until a toothpick inserted into the center comes out clean.

7. Let cool in the muffin tin for 10 minutes before transferring to a wire rack to cool completely.

Nutrition Information (per muffin):

- Calories: 140
- Protein: 4g
- Carbohydrates: 8g
- Fat: 11g
- Fiber: 3g
- Sugar: 2g
- Portion size: 1 muffin

# Raspberry Almond Tart

Ingredients:

- 1 cup almond flour
- 1/4 cup coconut flour
- 1/4 cup keto-friendly sweetener
- 1/4 cup melted butter
- 1/2 tsp almond extract
- 1/2 cup sugar-free raspberry jam

Instructions:

1. Preheat oven to 350°F (175°C). Grease a tart pan.
2. In a bowl, mix almond flour, coconut flour, sweetener, melted butter, and almond extract until crumbly.
3. Press mixture into the bottom and up the sides of the tart pan.
4. Bake for 12-15 minutes until golden brown.
5. Let cool completely before spreading raspberry jam over the crust.
6. Refrigerate for at least 1 hour before slicing and serving.

Nutrition Information (per serving - 1 slice):

- Calories: 160
- Protein: 4g
- Carbohydrates: 9g
- Fat: 12g

- Fiber: 3g
- Sugar: 1g
- Portion size: 1 slice

## Low Carb Chocolate Bark

Ingredients:

- 1 cup dark chocolate chips (sugar-free or at least 85% cocoa)
- 1/4 cup chopped nuts (almonds, walnuts, or pecans)
- 2 tbsp unsweetened shredded coconut
- Pinch of sea salt

Instructions:

1. Line a baking sheet with parchment paper.
2. Melt dark chocolate chips in a microwave-safe bowl in 30-second intervals, stirring in between until smooth.
3. Pour melted chocolate onto the parchment paper and spread evenly with a spatula.
4. Sprinkle chopped nuts, shredded coconut, and sea salt evenly over the chocolate.
5. Place in the refrigerator for 1 hour or until firm.
6. Break into pieces before serving.

Nutrition Information (per serving - 1 ounce):

- Calories: 120
- Protein: 2g
- Carbohydrates: 10g
- Fat: 9g
- Fiber: 3g
- Sugar: 1g
- Portion size: 1 ounce

## Peanut Butter Cups

Ingredients:

- 1/2 cup sugar-free chocolate chips
- 1/4 cup natural peanut butter (no added sugar)
- 2 tbsp coconut oil, divided

Instructions:

1. Line a mini muffin tin with paper liners.
2. Melt half of the chocolate chips with 1 tbsp of coconut oil in a microwave-safe bowl in 30-second intervals until smooth.
3. Spoon chocolate mixture into the bottom of each muffin liner, about 1 teaspoon per cup.
4. Place in the freezer for 10 minutes to set.

5. Meanwhile, melt peanut butter with remaining coconut oil until smooth.

6. Remove muffin tin from freezer and spoon peanut butter mixture over the chocolate layer, about 1 teaspoon per cup.

7. Melt remaining chocolate chips with coconut oil until smooth. Spoon over peanut butter layer to cover completely.

8. Place in the freezer for another 20 minutes until firm.

9. Remove paper liners before serving.

Nutrition Information (per serving - 2 peanut butter cups):

- Calories: 150
- Protein: 4g
- Carbohydrates: 8g
- Fat: 12g
- Fiber: 3g
- Sugar: 1g
- Portion size: 2 peanut butter cups

## Blueberry Muffins

Ingredients:

- 1 cup almond flour
- 1/4 cup coconut flour
- 1/4 cup keto-friendly sweetener

- 1 tsp baking powder

- 1/4 tsp salt

- 1/4 cup melted coconut oil

- 2 large eggs

- 1/4 cup unsweetened almond milk

- 1 tsp vanilla extract

- 1/2 cup fresh or frozen blueberries

Instructions:

1. Preheat oven to 350°F (175°C). Line a muffin tin with paper liners.

2. In a bowl, whisk together almond flour, coconut flour, sweetener, baking powder, and salt.

3. In another bowl, mix melted coconut oil, eggs, almond milk, and vanilla extract until smooth.

4. Combine wet and dry ingredients until well incorporated.

5. Gently fold in blueberries.

6. Spoon batter into muffin tin, filling each about 3/4 full.

7. Bake for 20-25 minutes or until a toothpick inserted into the center comes out clean.

8. Let cool in the muffin tin for 10 minutes before transferring to a wire rack to cool completely.

Nutrition Information (per muffin):

- Calories: 140
- Protein: 5g
- Carbohydrates: 7g
- Fat: 11g
- Fiber: 3g
- Sugar: 2g
- Portion size: 1 muffin

## Coconut Macaroons

Ingredients:

- 2 cups unsweetened shredded coconut
- 1/4 cup coconut flour
- 1/2 cup keto-friendly sweetener
- 1/4 cup melted coconut oil
- 2 large eggs
- 1 tsp vanilla extract
- Pinch of salt

Instructions:

1. Preheat oven to 325°F (160°C). Line a baking sheet with parchment paper.

2. In a bowl, mix shredded coconut, coconut flour, sweetener, and salt.

3. In another bowl, whisk melted coconut oil, eggs, and vanilla extract until well combined.

4. Combine wet and dry ingredients until a sticky dough forms.

5. Scoop tablespoon-sized portions of dough onto the baking sheet.

6. Bake for 18-20 minutes or until edges are golden brown.

7. Let cool completely on the baking sheet before serving.

Nutrition Information (per serving - 2 macaroons):

- Calories: 160
- Protein: 3g
- Carbohydrates: 7g
- Fat: 13g
- Fiber: 4g
- Sugar: 2g
- Portion size: 2 macaroons

## Chocolate Covered Strawberries

Ingredients:

- 1 cup sugar-free dark chocolate chips
- 1 tbsp coconut oil

- 15 large strawberries, washed and dried

Instructions:

1. Line a baking sheet with parchment paper.
2. In a microwave-safe bowl, melt dark chocolate chips with coconut oil in 30-second intervals until smooth.
3. Hold each strawberry by the stem and dip into the melted chocolate, coating about two-thirds of the berry.
4. Place each chocolate-covered strawberry on the prepared baking sheet.
5. Refrigerate for 30 minutes or until the chocolate sets.
6. Serve chilled.

Nutrition Information (per serving - 2 strawberries):

- Calories: 100
- Protein: 1g
- Carbohydrates: 10g
- Fat: 7g
- Fiber: 3g
- Sugar: 5g
- Portion size: 2 strawberries

# Chapter 7: Smoothies

Smoothies are a refreshing and nutritious way to start your day or enjoy as a snack. Packed with vitamins, minerals, and antioxidants, these recipes are designed to support your health goals while satisfying your taste buds. Each smoothie is easy to prepare and can be customized to suit your preferences.

## Green Detox Smoothie

Ingredients:

- 1 cup spinach
- 1/2 cup cucumber, peeled and chopped
- 1/2 green apple, chopped
- 1/2 lemon, juiced
- 1/2 inch fresh ginger, peeled
- 1/2 cup coconut water or water
- Ice cubes (optional)

Instructions:

1. Combine all ingredients in a blender.
2. Blend until smooth.
3. Serve immediately.

Nutrition Information:

- Calories: 90
- Protein: 2g
- Carbohydrates: 21g
- Fat: 0.5g
- Fiber: 4g
- Sugar: 12g
- Portion size: 1 serving

## Berry Blast Smoothie

Ingredients:

- 1 cup mixed berries (strawberries, blueberries, raspberries)
- 1/2 cup plain Greek yogurt
- 1/2 cup almond milk
- 1 tablespoon honey or maple syrup (optional)
- Ice cubes (optional)

Instructions:

1. Place all ingredients in a blender.
2. Blend until smooth and creamy.
3. Pour into a glass and serve.

Nutrition Information:

- Calories: 150
- Protein: 8g
- Carbohydrates: 25g
- Fat: 2g
- Fiber: 5g
- Sugar: 18g
- Portion size: 1 serving

## Avocado Spinach Smoothie

Ingredients:

- 1/2 ripe avocado
- 1 cup fresh spinach
- 1/2 cup pineapple chunks
- 1/2 cup coconut water or almond milk
- Juice of 1/2 lime
- Ice cubes (optional)

Instructions:

1. Combine all ingredients in a blender.
2. Blend until smooth and creamy.
3. Serve immediately.

Nutrition Information:

- Calories: 180
- Protein: 3g
- Carbohydrates: 25g
- Fat: 9g
- Fiber: 7g
- Sugar: 13g
- Portion size: 1 serving

## Coconut Almond Smoothie

Ingredients:

- 1/2 cup coconut milk
- 1/2 cup almond milk
- 1 tablespoon almond butter
- 1 tablespoon shredded coconut
- 1 teaspoon honey or maple syrup (optional)
- Ice cubes (optional)

Instructions:

1. Blend all ingredients until smooth.
2. Pour into a glass and enjoy.

Nutrition Information:

- Calories: 220
- Protein: 5g
- Carbohydrates: 10g
- Fat: 18g
- Fiber: 3g
- Sugar: 5g
- Portion size: 1 serving

## Tropical Mango Smoothie

Ingredients:

- 1 cup frozen mango chunks
- 1/2 cup pineapple chunks
- 1/2 cup plain Greek yogurt
- 1/2 cup coconut water or water
- Ice cubes (optional)

Instructions:

1. Combine all ingredients in a blender.
2. Blend until smooth and creamy.
3. Serve immediately.

Nutrition Information:

- Calories: 200
- Protein: 10g
- Carbohydrates: 35g
- Fat: 1g
- Fiber: 4g
- Sugar: 30g
- Portion size: 1 serving

## Chocolate Peanut Butter Smoothie

Ingredients:

- 1 banana, frozen
- 1 tablespoon cocoa powder
- 1 tablespoon peanut butter
- 1 cup almond milk
- Ice cubes (optional)

Instructions:

1. Blend all ingredients until smooth.
2. Pour into a glass and serve.

Nutrition Information:

- Calories: 250

- Protein: 7g

- Carbohydrates: 30g

- Fat: 13g

- Fiber: 7g

- Sugar: 15g

- Portion size: 1 serving


## Strawberry Banana Smoothie

Ingredients:

- 1 cup strawberries, fresh or frozen

- 1 banana

- 1/2 cup plain Greek yogurt

- 1/2 cup almond milk

- Ice cubes (optional)


Instructions:

1. Combine all ingredients in a blender.

2. Blend until smooth and creamy.

3. Serve immediately.


Nutrition Information:

- Calories: 180

- Protein: 9g

- Carbohydrates: 30g
- Fat: 3g
- Fiber: 5g
- Sugar: 18g
- Portion size: 1 serving

## Blueberry Kale Smoothie

Ingredients:

- 1 cup blueberries, fresh or frozen
- 1 cup chopped kale leaves
- 1/2 cup plain Greek yogurt
- 1/2 cup almond milk
- 1 tablespoon honey or maple syrup (optional)
- Ice cubes (optional)

Instructions:

1. Blend all ingredients until smooth.
2. Pour into a glass and enjoy.

Nutrition Information:

- Calories: 160
- Protein: 9g
- Carbohydrates: 30g

- Fat: 2g

- Fiber: 6g

- Sugar: 20g

- Portion size: 1 serving

## Cinnamon Vanilla Smoothie

Ingredients:

- 1 banana, frozen

- 1/2 teaspoon ground cinnamon

- 1/2 teaspoon vanilla extract

- 1/2 cup plain Greek yogurt

- 1/2 cup almond milk

- Ice cubes (optional)

Instructions:

1. Blend all ingredients until smooth.

2. Pour into a glass and serve.

Nutrition Information:

- Calories: 200

- Protein: 10g

- Carbohydrates: 35g

- Fat: 3g

- Fiber: 5g

- Sugar: 20g

- Portion size: 1 serving

## Raspberry Lemonade Smoothie

Ingredients:

- 1 cup raspberries, fresh or frozen

- Juice of 1 lemon

- 1/2 cup plain Greek yogurt

- 1/2 cup coconut water or water

- 1 tablespoon honey or maple syrup (optional)

- Ice cubes (optional)

Instructions:

1. Combine all ingredients in a blender.

2. Blend until smooth and creamy.

3. Serve immediately.

Nutrition Information:

- Calories: 160

- Protein: 8g

- Carbohydrates: 30g

- Fat: 2g

- Fiber: 6g

- Sugar: 20g

- Portion size: 1 serving

## Mint Chocolate Smoothie

Ingredients:

- 1 cup spinach

- 1/2 cup fresh mint leaves

- 1 tablespoon cocoa powder

- 1/2 banana, frozen

- 1/2 cup almond milk

- Ice cubes (optional)

Instructions:

1. Blend all ingredients until smooth.

2. Pour into a glass and enjoy.

Nutrition Information:

- Calories: 150

- Protein: 5g

- Carbohydrates: 25g

- Fat: 5g

- Fiber: 6g

- Sugar: 12g

- Portion size: 1 serving

# Pumpkin Pie Smoothie

Ingredients:

- 1/2 cup pumpkin puree

- 1/2 banana, frozen

- 1/2 teaspoon pumpkin pie spice

- 1/2 cup plain Greek yogurt

- 1/2 cup almond milk

- Ice cubes (optional)

Instructions:

1. Blend all ingredients until smooth.

2. Pour into a glass and serve.

Nutrition Information:

- Calories: 180

- Protein: 9g

- Carbohydrates: 30g

- Fat: 3g

- Fiber: 6g

- Sugar: 15g

- Portion size: 1 serving

## Matcha Green Tea Smoothie

Ingredients:

- 1 teaspoon matcha powder
- 1 banana, frozen
- 1/2 cup spinach
- 1/2 cup plain Greek yogurt
- 1/2 cup almond milk
- Ice cubes (optional)

Instructions:

1. Blend all ingredients until smooth.
2. Pour into a glass and enjoy.

Nutrition Information:

- Calories: 180
- Protein: 9g
- Carbohydrates: 30g
- Fat: 3g
- Fiber: 5g
- Sugar: 18g
- Portion size: 1 serving

# Almond Butter and Jelly Smoothie

Ingredients:

- 1/2 cup mixed berries (strawberries, blueberries, raspberries)
- 1 tablespoon almond butter
- 1/2 cup plain Greek yogurt
- 1/2 cup almond milk
- Ice cubes (optional)

Instructions:

1. Blend all ingredients until smooth.
2. Pour into a glass and serve.

Nutrition Information:

- Calories: 200
- Protein: 10g
- Carbohydrates: 25g
- Fat: 8g
- Fiber: 5g
- Sugar: 18g
- Portion size: 1 serving

# Pineapple Ginger Smoothie

Ingredients:

- 1 cup pineapple chunks
- 1/2 inch fresh ginger, peeled
- 1/2 cup plain Greek yogurt
- 1/2 cup coconut water or water
- Ice cubes (optional)

Instructions:

1. Combine all ingredients in a blender.
2. Blend until smooth and creamy.
3. Serve immediately.

Nutrition Information:

- Calories: 180
- Protein: 9g
- Carbohydrates: 35g
- Fat: 1g
- Fiber: 3g
- Sugar: 28g
- Portion size: 1 serving

# CONCLUSION

Congratulations on completing "Low Carb Vegetarian Type 2 Diabetes Cookbooks for Beginners"! This book has been crafted with your health and well-being in mind, offering a wealth of delicious recipes tailored to manage Type 2 diabetes through a low carb vegetarian diet.

Throughout this journey, you've explored diverse flavors and creative cooking techniques that prove managing diabetes doesn't mean sacrificing taste or variety. By focusing on nutrient-dense ingredients and balanced meal planning, you've equipped yourself with powerful tools to maintain stable blood sugar levels and promote overall health.

Remember, this book is just the beginning of your culinary adventure. As you continue on your path, embrace the joy of experimenting with new dishes and ingredients. Stay curious and open to discovering what works best for you and your body.

Always keep in mind the importance of consistency and moderation in your diet. Whether you're enjoying a hearty breakfast, a satisfying lunch, or a delightful dessert, each recipe has been thoughtfully designed to support your journey towards better health.

As you move forward, don't hesitate to revisit the meal plans, adapt recipes to suit your preferences, and explore additional resources provided. Your commitment to a healthy lifestyle is commendable, and every step you take brings you closer to achieving your wellness goals.

Thank you for choosing "Low Carb Vegetarian Type 2 Diabetes Cookbooks for Beginners". May your kitchen continue to be a place of nourishment, joy, and empowerment. Here's to your health and happiness!

Remember, your health is your greatest wealth.